Healing Poultices

Healing Poultices

**By Monica Sidoine,
S.N.H.S. Dip. Herbalism**

DISCLAIMER

This book is to serve as an informational guide for use in the home. The remedies and procedures contained in this book are meant to supplement and are not intended to be a substitute for professional medical care. Please seek a qualified medical practitioner for all ailments. The author nor distributors takes no responsibility for customers choosing to treat themselves. Your use of this information is at your own risk.

ISBN - 13: 978-1534889774
ISBN - 10: 1534889779

Proof Read by Jasmine Ned Anunda

Printed By Create Space Publishing
United States of America

ACKNOWLEDGMENTS

I would like to thank all those who have contributed in one way or another to the completion of "HEALING POULTICES."

I thank God for giving me the vision, wisdom and good health to write this book. For all he has done and will continue to do in my life.

For the many prayer warriors who interceded on behalf of this project and also their moral support.

I thank my daughter Jasmine Ned Anunda for proof reading.

Thank you all.

Monica Sidoine.

PREFACE

And Isaiah said, Take a lump of figs. And they took and laid it on the boil, and he recovered. 2 Kings 20:7 (KJV)

When he had thus spoken, he spat on the ground, and made clay of the spittle, and he anointed the eyes of the blind man with the clay.

And said unto him, Go, wash in the pool of Si-lo-am, (Which is by interpretation, Sent.) He went his way therefore, and washed, and came seeing. John 9:6 & 7 (KJV)

In the midst of the street of it, and on either side of the river, was there the tree of life, which bare twelve manner of fruits, and yielded her fruit every month; and the leaves of the tree were for the healing of the nations. Revelation 22:2 (KJV)

Poultices were being used in Bible times and they brought healing. They are currently being used and they still bring healing.

The procedures in this Book was designed to be as simple as possible so that anyone will be able to follow them. Most of the items used are local things which you would either have at home, in your cupboard or kitchen garden; or you might be able to get it from a friend; if not they can be easily purchased from the local market or health store for a low cost.

The poultices presented in this book are very healing and useful. I, family and friends have used some of these poultices and we have received healing as a result. It is my wish that they would be of great benefit to you and others.

TABLE OF CONTENTS

POULTICES

A poultice is a cold or warm moist preparation placed on a wound, an aching or inflamed part of the body.

It is used to assist with the following:-

To adsorb.

To ease pain and congestion.

To improve circulation.

To reduce inflammation.

To ease tension and swelling.

To relax the muscles.

Stings and insect bites.

To hasten the expression of pus.

To draw impurities out through the skin.

To promote absorption of poisons.

To soothe irritation.

To deodorize.

As an antiseptic and disinfectant.

Method:

Bruise an herb leaf and apply it to the skin.

Or mix dried cut or powdered herbs together.
Add water or some other liquid to it to form a paste.
Oats or grind flaxseed can also be added to bind it if needs be.
Apply it to the skin then cover or bandage the area.

It can also be applied between 2 layers of gauze or light cotton, then cover with a bandage. The poultice should be large enough to cover the area being treated.

Change it nightly and daily. The one that you would put on in the morning, remove it in the night and put on a fresh to leave on overnight to be changed in the morning.

After removing it wipe the area with a cold moist cloth.

A Cold Poultice is used to draw heat and inflammation from an inflamed and congested area.

A Hot Poultice is used to ease spasm and pain.

When using a Poultice on a hole in the body or a deep wound:

Clean and disinfect the area first. Add some anti-infection herbs to the poultice such as goldenseal, garlic, or tea tree oil. Once the poultice is dried it may look like some of it is gone or has been absorbed into the body; don't clean the remaining poultice off unless you need to recheck the wound. Just add a new poultice over the old one and keep feeding the area.

Categories of Poultices:

Herb Poultices:
Fenugreek, neem, sage, comfrey, arnica, etc.

Fruit Poultices:
Bananas, figs, apples, papayas and melons.

Vegetable Poultices:
Potatoes, onions, carrots, beets, garlic, cucumbers and a wide variety of greens.

Seed and Grain Poultices:
Oats, barley, flaxseed, etc.
They have very soothing effects.

Heating and Stimulating Poultices:
Cayenne, ginger, mustard and horseradish.

Healing and Soothing Poultices:
Slippery Elm, marshmallow, aloes, calendula, lobelia and mullein.

Drawing Poultice:
Charcoal.
It removes impurities and poisons out of the body and can be more effective if changed 1- 3 times a day.

Some Useful Poultices

Avocado Poultice:
Boil mashed avocado seeds with some water till it gets to a light paste.
It is good for furuncles and abscesses.

Bread Poultice:
Warm 1 tablespoon milk and pour it over a slice of bread.
Mash to a paste.
Apply it to the warm to the area allowing it to dry. Do it twice daily.
It is good for boils, infections and for removing splinters.

Cabbage Poultice:
Crush or grate the leaves and lay it on the skin.
Some flaxseed or oats can be added to help bind the grated one.
Put a cloth bandage on it. When it feels hot, replace it with a fresh one or it can be applied nightly and changed in the morning with a fresh one.
This will draw out poisons and pus, eczema, acne, furuncles, infected wounds, varicose and torpid ulcers, very good for strains, sprains, swellings and broken bones.
For arthritis boil the cabbage leaves, cook slightly. Apply it warm to the hands and joints.

Calendula Poultice:
Wrap some fresh flower petals in a fine cotton cloth.
Apply it to the area.
It is good for skin sores, eczema, burns, furuncles, wounds and joint pains.

Carrot Poultice #1:
Grate the carrots fine and soak it or use the pulp after juicing.
Apply it to the wound.
It is very good for sore congested painful parts, also mastitis - breast inflammation, bruises, sores, chapped skin and nipples.

Carrot Poultice #2:
Boil the carrot and mash it.
It is good for infected wounds, burns, acne, eczema, abscesses and also to soothe the skin.

Cassava Poultice:
Add some lemon juice to some cassava flour.
Apply the poultice hot to the area.
It is good for furuncles, abscesses and infected sores.

Castor Bean Leaf Poultice:
Take 12 fresh leaves and crush them.
Moisten with a little warm water.
Very good for wounds, eczema, herpes, burns, skin rashes and hair loss.

Cayenne Poultice:
Heat 1 part coconut oil until hot.
Mix 1 part cayenne pepper with it to form a paste. Cool.
Apply to the skin and keep in place with a bandage.
During the day add more coconut oil if necessary to keep it moist.
Reapply every day.
Will relieve pain, stiffness in the neck, muscular aches, rheumatism, reduces congestion of the internal organs and tissues, reduce swelling and speed healing.

Charcoal Poultice:
Mix powdered charcoal in a little water to the thickness of a paste.

Some ground flaxseed or oats can be added to help bind it.
Spread it on a piece of cotton cloth or folded paper towel.
Put it on the area, cover with a piece of plastic and tape or bandage it.
Leave it on overnight and remove in the morning.
Sponge the area with cold water or rub gently with a cold cloth.
It may be placed over a boil or an area of dermatitis, poison ivy, insect stings, ulcers, wounds and over the kidney area for kidney disease etc.
It can be placed over the abdomen to treat diarrhea.
A layer of charcoal can be sprinkled on the surface of ulcers and infected wounds.

Chickweed Poultice:
Boil 4oz in ½ liter of water until it forms a paste.
Apply it to the area.
It is good for inflammation of the skin due to sunburn, bruises and irritations.

Clay and Glycerin Poultice:
Dig up some clay several inches from the earth's surface. Make sure that it is fine and free from any other thing.
Sterilize it in the oven at 350°F for a few minutes to make sure that it is properly heated. Add some water and a few tablespoons of glycerin to get it moist.
Apply it to the area. Cover with a few layers of cotton cloth.
It can be left on for at least 6 hours. Rinse and dry the area.
It is very good for skin rashes and skin diseases.

It can also be used as a face mask by applying a thin layer which will help to improve the blood circulation and remove impurities.

Clay Poultice:
Mix some clay with water to make a paste.
Apply it to the area. Cover with a few layers of cotton cloth.

It can be left on for at least 6 hours but constantly apply water on it to keep it moist. Rinse and dry the area.

It is very good for reducing inflammation, increased blood circulation, drawing out pus and infections from wounds, skin rashes and skin diseases. It can be applied over the liver area to improve the function of the liver and also for detoxification.

Cocoa Poultice:

Roast 10 cocoa seeds and pound them very fine.

Apply it to the area after taking a warm bath.

It is good for athlete foot fungus.

Comfrey Poultice:

Crush the leaves and moisten with some comfrey tea.

Apply it to the area.

It is good for wounds, open sores, ulcers, burns, eczema, rash, skin irritations and inflammations, and swellings.

Cornmeal Poultice:

Steep 1oz of corn hair in1 liter of boiling water for 20 minutes.

Add 4 cups of cornmeal to make a paste.

Apply it hot over the bladder or kidney at bedtime or for 10 minutes three times daily.

Very good for the kidney and inflammation of the bladder.

Fenugreek Poultice:

Boil 4oz of ground fenugreek seeds in 1 liter of water for 15 minutes.

Place it on a cloth and apply it over the affected part.

For hemorrhoids apply it cold on the anus.

For these cases apply it hot – ulcers, wounds which take long to heal, nipple and lip cracks, arthritis, joint rheumatism, inflamed or aching joints.

Figs Poultice:
Boil some figs in a small amount of water for 5 minutes. Cut open. Apply the hot figs on the area. Very good for boils, infected sores, furuncles, abscesses, tumors and skin inflammation.
A mashed hot leaf can also be applied on a wart.

Flaxseed Poultice:
Grind 1 tablespoon of flaxseed, mix it with 1 cup of boiling water. Stir briskly with a wooden spoon.
This makes enough paste to cover the front of the abdomen.
Spread the mixture on a piece of damp cloth, over a paper towel or directly on the skin. Cover with a larger piece of plastic, hold in place with a strip of cloth or a bandage.
Leave it on for 30 minutes to 8 hours or overnight.
Remove it, wash the area with a washcloth, and then give a cold mitten friction, dry thoroughly.
It is very good for painful areas, insect bites, colds, bronchitis, menstrual pain, intestinal spasms, abscesses, furuncles, kidney and gallbladder pains.

Garlic Poultice #1:
Crush fresh garlic and add warm water and flour just enough to bind the garlic.
Place it on a cloth then over the affected part.
It hurts when left on too long, as soon as the part hurts remove it.
It is very effective when applied to the reflexology areas on the foot corresponding to the infected part of the body.
Used to neutralize the acids. It is an antiseptic and antibacterial preparation. It relieves pain, infection and pus. It is good for fungus skin infection, boils, eczema, dermatitis, arthritis and to reduce abscesses.

Garlic Poultice #2:
Crush some garlic cloves very fine.
Add a little finely grated ginger or a pinch of cayenne powder to it.
Moisten it with a little hot water.
Apply it to the skin. Put a moist hot washcloth over it, then a dry cloth.
Very good for measles and chicken pox.

Hops Poultice:
Crush the leaves and moisten them with some hot water.
Put it on a folded paper towel. Apply it to the area.
It is good for boils, bruises, toothaches, earaches, ulcers, skin infections, rheumatic pains and inflammation.

Wrap a handful of hop cones in a cotton cloth. Soak it in warm water. Apply it over the aching area.
It is good for stomach aches and neuralgic pain.

Mustard Plaster:
Mix 1 tablespoon of dry mustard to 4 tablespoons of wheat flour for an adult, 1 tablespoon mustard to 8 tablespoons flour for a child, 1 tablespoon mustard to 12 tablespoons flour for an infant. Add enough lukewarm water to make a thin paste.
Spread it on a cloth and fold over. Place a thin cotton cloth over the effected part. Put on the poultice, then a large piece of plastic to cover it and a towel. A warm towel or hot water bottle can be applied over this to increase the heat.
Leave it on for 20 minutes. Remove it earlier if it is burning, stinging or the skin has become well reddened. Wipe the area with a cloth or paper tissue dipped in vegetable oil to remove the mustard. Cover the area with a warm blanket and leave on overnight.
Very good for backache, circulation and pain in arthritic joints.
When olive oil is added it is good for easing congestion of a part.

Neem Poultice:
Coarsely grind 1lb neem leaves and 4oz neem bark and mix them in a blender.
Place in a sealed container. Mix 1 cup of the mixture with hot water and stir until it is wet. Cool. Place in a nylon bag and secure it to the wound with a cotton cloth.
Leave it on for several hours. Repeat daily as needed.
Very good for muscle sprains, pain, bruises or skin wounds and also diabetics with slow healing wounds.

Noni Poultice:
Crush noni leaves and moisten with a little warm water.
Apply it over the affected areas and cover with a dry cloth.
Very good for wounds and pain.

Oatmeal Poultice:
Cook oatmeal, cool then place it in a soft cotton cloth.
Apply it over the affected areas and cover with a dry cloth.
Apply a heating pad or a warm cloth over it.
It is very good for insect bites, wounds, cuts and eczema.
It's a general anti-inflammatory poultice.

Onion Poultice:
Grate or chop the onion into small pieces.
Put it on a thin cotton cloth and fold.
Place it on the chest or under the soles of the feet.
Place it on the forehead for sinus headaches.
Put it on the bladder area for bladder inflammation.
Check every 30 minutes for skin irritation.
Very good for bruises, injuries and inflamed areas.

Parsley Poultice:
Chop fresh parsley leaves. Moisten with a little hot water.

Put it in a thin cotton cloth and fold, put it on the area when it has cooled down a bit.
Very good for insect bites, bruises and rheumatism.

Plantain Poultice:
Boil the leaves then mash them.
Rub the affected area with uncooked leaves, then apply the poultice.
It is good for insect bites.
For a swollen or running sore apply a crushed leaf to it.

Potato Poultice:
Grate and soak the potato.
Apply it to the area and cover with a cotton cloth.
It is very good for itching, burning sensations, bruises, sprains, boils and black eye.

Prickly Pear Poultice:
Splice the leaves open. Heat them lightly for a few minutes.
Apply on the affected are.
It is very good for skin irritations, wounds and bruises.

Psyllium Seed Poultice:
Mash the seeds and steep them for 1 hour. Heat the seeds.
Apply the poultice to the affected are for 15 minutes three times daily.
It is good for skin infections, burns, wounds and varicose ulceration.

Red Clover Poultice:
Boil some seeds, mash them and add a little warm water to make a paste.
It is very good for burns, wounds and abscesses.

Rice Poultice:
Soak some rice in a small amount of water for 1 hour.
Strain and crush the rice into a paste.

Apply to the area and cover with a cotton cloth.
Very good for wounds.

Rosemary Poultice:
Mix 4oz of ground linseed with 10 drops of rosemary oil.
Apply it to the area and cover with a towel.
Leave it on for 15 minutes. Do it twice daily till better, then once daily.
It is very good for rheumatism.

Sage Poultice:
Crush fresh sage leaves and moisten with a little warm water or use the tea.
It is very good for injuries, painful grazes and abrasions.

Salt Poultice:
Heat 1-2lbs of coarse salt. Put it in a small cushion case.
Apply it to the injured or painful area.

Soap Poultice:
Mix together equal amounts of grated bar soap and sugar till it gets like a paste. If the bar soap is moist you can just cut off a piece and work the sugar into it. Heat it for just 1 or 2 minutes.
Apply it warm over the entire area. Cover it with a bandage.
Leave it on for at least 20 hours.
Wipe the area. It can be repeated.
Good for boils, abscesses and removing splinters.

Sorrel Poultice:
Crush sorrel leaves and moisten with a little warm water.
It is good for acne and skin blemishes.

Soursop Poultice:
Crush soursop leaves and moisten with a little warm water.

It is very good for mumps and skin infections.
Apply it below the ear for mumps.

Thyme Poultice:
Moisten some thyme with a little hot water.
Wrap it in a thin cotton cloth and put it on the bruise when it has cooled down a bit.
It is good for arthritis, gout, sciatica, lumbalgia and stiff neck pains.

Turmeric Poultice:
Mix 1 teaspoon of grated turmeric with a little water into a paste.
Spread it on a cotton cloth and fold. Put it on the boils, put a bandage or tape on it.

This is good for boils but can also be used for pain and inflammation but ½ teaspoon of ginger or cayenne and more turmeric will have to be added.

Watercress Poultice:
Crush some watercress and wrap it in a thin cotton cloth.
Put it on the area.
It enhances and regenerate the skin in these cases - eczema, acne, dermatosis, wounds and sores.

INDEX

Other Book Titles by the Same Author

Can be viewed at this link:
http://www.amazon.com/author/monicasidoine

Home Remedies For Cancer

Home Remedies For Losing Weight

Home Remedies For Blood Pressure and Diabetes

Home Remedies For Headaches and Insomnia

Home Remedies For Sinusitis and Tonsillitis

Home Remedies For Constipation and Diarrhea

Home Remedies For Asthma and Bronchitis

Home Remedies For Dehydration and Vomiting

Home Remedies For Pneumonia and Tuberculosis

Home Remedies For Stress, Depression and Anxiety

Home Remedies For Colds, Fever and Sore Throat

Home Remedies For Heart Attack and Strokes

The 20 Most Valuable Herbs

NOTES

NOTES

NOTES

NOTES

www.ingramcontent.com/pod-product-compliance
Lightning Source LLC
Chambersburg PA
CBHW061945280526
45787CB00004B/1733